# YOU HAVE LUPUS NOW WHAT?
# BY
# PATTI CHIAPPA

Copyright © 2017 Dark Starlight Publications/ Patti Chiappa

All rights reserved. No part of this publication may be reproduced, distributed, or transmitted in any form or by any means, including photocopying, recording, or other electronic or mechanical methods, without the prior written permission of the publisher, except in the case of brief quotations

EMBODIED IN CRITICAL REVIEWS AND CERTAIN OTHER NONCOMMERCIAL USES PERMITTED BY COPYRIGHT LAW. FRIST EDITION PRINTED IN THE U.S. A. PLEASE NOTE: THIS BOOK WAS WRITTEN BY SOMEONE WHO HAS A LEARNING DISABILITY, TRAUMATIC BRAIN INJURY AND MUST OF ALL I AM A VICTIM OF LUPUS ALSO. (TBI) IS A FORM OF BRAIN INJURY CAUSED BY SUDDEN DAMAGE TO THE BRAIN. (I GOT MINE FROM HAVING TWO STROKES) I SHARE THIS WITH YOU NOT TO GAIN YOUR

SYMPATHY BUT TO SHARE AND INSPIRE THAT PEOPLE WITH DISABILITIES CAN DO ANYTHING THEY SET THEIR MIND TO.

THIS BOOK IS NOT INTENDED AS A SUBSTITUTE FOR THE MEDICAL ADVICE OF PHYSICIANS. THE READER SHOULD REGULARLY CONSULT A PHYSICIAN IN MATTERS RELATING TO HIS/HER HEALTH AND PARTICULARLY WITH RESPECT TO ANY SYMPTOMS THAT MAY REQUIRE DIAGNOSIS OR MEDICAL ATTENTION.

**I AM NOT A MEDICAL PROFESSIONAL. THIS BOOK WAS WRITTEN TO SHARE MY OWN EXPERIENCE WITH LUPUS AND NOTHING CAN REPLACE A DOCTOR!**

# Introduction

My name is Patricia Ann Chiappa. But you can call me Patti for short. In Oct of 2000, I started to become ill. My symptoms ranged from me passing out to getting a painful rash all over my body, that doctors diagnosed as hives to feeling very tired. I went to many doctors, who ran many tests from EKGs to blood tests. They couldn't come with a cause. So, they said it was all in my mind.

They sent me to a shrink. They said I was under stress and having a mental breakdown. But I wasn't! I just had lupus. Lupus that cause me to have two major strokes, four miscarriages, a host of other illnesses including a brain injury, blood clots and fibromyalgia.

I was finally diagnosed with lupus, after my medical doctor gave me a simple blood test called an antinuclear

ANTIBODY (ANA) TEST. THAT TURNED OUT TO BE POSITIVE. THAT ALONG WITH ALL MY SYMPTOMS CONFIRMED I WAS NOT MENTALLY ILL, BUT HAD A MISUNDERSTOOD ILLNESS. IT TOOK MY DOCTORS A LONG 17 YEARS TO FIND OUT I HAD LUPUS. IN THIS BOOK YOU WILL FIND TREATMENTS FOR LUPUS, LUPUS DIET, SYMPTOMS, WHAT BLOOD TESTS YOU NEED TO TAKE TO FIND OUT YOU HAVE LUPUS, AND MUCH MORE.

## "What is Lupus? Chapter 1"

Lupus is a complicated condition; there are different types and people often show different symptoms on different parts of the body. As such it's often misunderstood by the public.

The term lupus will refer to systemic lupus erythematosus ~ or SLE ~ which is one of the more serious forms of the condition.

SLE can exhibit different symptoms, and some people will experience them more severely than others. The most common are fatigue, swollen or painful joints, and skin irritation or rashes, particularly around the hands, wrists or face.

Other symptoms can include a fever, swollen glands, headaches or migraines, and stomach pains. Of course, these can be caused by many issues, so it's important that you speak to your doctor who'll be able to make a diagnosis.

Other types of lupus will just affect the skin.

SLE is an autoimmune condition, meaning it's not contagious and can't be passed from one person to another. Instead, it's caused when antibodies from the immune system mistakenly attack

HEALTHY CELLS OR ORGANS.

EXPERTS STILL AREN'T ENTIRELY CERTAIN WHY THIS HAPPENS, THE CONDITION CAN ALSO BE AFFECTED BY CHANGES IN HORMONES, FROM PREGNANCY OR PUBERTY FOR EXAMPLE, SO IT'S MOST PREVALENT IN WOMEN OF CHILDBEARING AGE.

WHILE THERE'S CURRENTLY NO CURE FOR SLE, THERE ARE MEDICATIONS AVAILABLE TO MANAGE ITS IMPACT SUCH AS ANTI-INFLAMMATORIES, OR MEDICINES THAT

SUPPRESS YOUR IMMUNE SYSTEM. BY USING THESE, MANY PEOPLE CAN SUCCESSFULLY MANAGE THE CONDITION TO LIMIT THE IMPACT THEIR DAY TO DAY LIVES.

## "Symptoms of Lupus- Chapter 2"

### 1. Fatigue

About 90 percent of people with lupus experience some level of fatigue. An afternoon nap does the trick for some people, but sleeping too much during the day can lead to insomnia at night. It may be difficult, but if you can remain active and stick to a daily routine, you may be able to keep your energy levels up.

## 2. Unexplained fever

One of the early symptoms of lupus is a low-grade fever for no apparent reason. Because it may hover somewhere between 98.5°F (36.9°C) and 101°F (38.3°C), you might not think to see a doctor. People with lupus may experience this type of fever off and on.

## 3. Hair loss

Thinning hair is often one of the first symptoms of lupus. Hair loss is the result of inflammation of the skin and scalp. Some people with lupus lose hair by the clump. More often, hair thins out slowly. Some people also have thinning of the beard, eyebrows, eyelashes, and other body hair. Lupus can cause hair to feel brittle, break easily, and look a bit ragged, earning it the name "lupus hair."

## 4. Skin Rash or Lesions

One of the most visible symptoms of lupus is a butterfly-shaped rash that appears over the bridge of the nose and on both cheeks. About 50 percent of people with lupus have this rash. It can occur suddenly or appear after exposure to sunlight. Sometimes the rash appears just before a flare-up.

Lupus can also cause non-itchy lesions in other areas of the body. Rarely, lupus can cause hives. Many people with lupus are sensitive to the sun, or even to artificial lighting. Some experience discoloration in the fingers and toes.

5. Pulmonary Issues

Inflammation of the pulmonary system is another possible symptom of lupus. The lungs become inflamed, and the swelling can extend to lung blood vessels. Even the diaphragm may be affected. These conditions can all lead to chest pain when you try to breathe in. This condition is often referred to as pleuritic chest pain.

Over time, breathing issues from lupus can shrink lung size. Ongoing chest pain and shortness of breath characterize this condition. It's sometimes called vanishing (or shrinking lung syndrome). The diaphragmatic muscles are so weak they appear to move up in CT scan images, according to the

Lupus Foundation of America.

## 6. Kidney Inflammation

People with lupus can develop a kidney inflammation called nephritis. Inflammation makes it harder for the kidneys to filter toxins and waste from the blood. According to the Lupus Foundation of America, nephritis usually begins within five years of the start of lupus.

## 7. Painful, Swollen Joints

Inflammation can cause pain, stiffness, and visible swelling in your joints, particularly in the morning. It may be mild at first and gradually become more obvious. Like other symptoms of lupus, joint problems can come and go.

If over-the-counter (OTC) pain medications don't help, see your doctor. There may be better treatment options. But your doctor must determine if your joint problems are caused by lupus or another condition, such as arthritis.

## 8. Gastrointestinal problems

Some people with lupus experience occasional heartburn, acid reflux, or other gastrointestinal problems. Mild symptoms can be treated with OTC antacids. If you have frequent bouts of acid reflux or heartburn, try cutting down on the size of your meals, and avoid beverages containing caffeine. Also, don't lie down right after a meal. If symptoms continue, see your doctor to rule out other conditions.

## 9. Thyroid Problems

It's not uncommon for people with lupus to develop autoimmune thyroid disease. The thyroid helps control your body's metabolism. A poorly functioning thyroid can affect vital organs like your brain, heart, kidneys, and liver. It can also result in weight gain or weight loss. Other symptoms include dry skin and hair, and moodiness.

When a thyroid is underactive, the condition is known as hypothyroidism. Hyperthyroidism is caused by an overactive thyroid. Treatments to get your metabolism back on track are available.

10. Dry Mouth, Dry Eyes

If you have lupus, you may experience dry mouth. Your eyes may feel gritty and dry, too. That's because some people with lupus develop Sjogren's disease, another autoimmune disorder. Sjogren's causes the glands responsible for tears and saliva to malfunction, and lymphocytes can accumulate in the glands. In some cases, women with lupus and Sjogren's may also experience dryness of the vagina and skin.

Central Nervous System - Lupus affects the brain or

central nervous system in some patients. Headaches, dizziness, memory disturbances, vision problems, seizures, stroke, or changes in behavior can result.

Blood Vessels - Blood vessels may become inflamed (vasculitis), affecting circulation. The inflammation may be mild or severe.

Blood - Lupus patients may develop anemia, leukopenia (a decreased number of white blood cells), or thrombocytopenia (a decrease in the number of platelets in the blood, which assist in clotting). Some people with lupus may have an increased risk for blood clots.

Heart - In some people with lupus, inflammation can affect the heart (myocarditis and endocarditis) or the membrane that surrounds it (pericarditis), causing chest pains or other symptoms. Lupus can also

Increase the risk of atherosclerosis (hardening of the arteries).

Nearly all patients with SLE report some symptoms relating to problems that occur in the central nervous system (CNS), which includes the spinal cord and the brain.

Symptoms vary widely and may overlap with psychiatric or neurologic disorders. They may also be caused by of some

# Medications used for treating SLE.

The most serious CNS disorder is inflammation of the blood vessels in the brain (CNS vasculitis), which occurs in about 10% of patients with SLE. Fever, seizures, psychosis, and even coma can occur. Other CNS side effects include:

Irritability

Emotional disorders (anxiety, depression)

Mild impairment of concentration and memory

Migraine and tension headaches

Problems with the reflex systems, sensation, vision, hearing, and motor control.

## Infections

Infections are a common complication and a major cause of death in all stages of SLE. Patients are not only prone to the ordinary bacterial and viral infections, but they are also susceptible to fungal and parasitic infections, which are common in people with weakened immune systems. They also face an increased risk for urinary tract, herpes, salmonella, and yeast infections. Corticosteroid and immunosuppressant drug treatments used for SLE also increase the risk for infections.

## Pregnancy Complications

Women with lupus face a higher risk for pregnancy complications, including miscarriage, premature birth, and preeclampsia. The risk for miscarriage is highest for patients with antiphospholipid antibodies, which can cause blood clotting in the placenta. Lupus patients with active kidney disease are at increased risk for preeclampsia (a pregnancy complication that includes high blood pressure and fluid build-up). Pregnant women who take corticosteroids face increased risks of gestational diabetes and high blood pressure.

You also might experience the following:

Osteoporosis

Cataracts

Glaucoma

Diabetes

Fluid retention

Susceptibility to infections

Weight gain

High blood pressure

Acne

Excess hair growth

Wasting of the muscles

# MENSTRUAL IRREGULARITIES
# IRRITABILITY
# INSOMNIA

# "What is the AMA Test- Chapter 3"

## Tests for Autoantibodies (ANA Test)

Antinuclear antibodies (ANAs). A primary test for SLE checks for antinuclear antibodies (ANA), which attack the cell nucleus.

High levels of ANA are found in more than 98% of patients with SLE. Other conditions, however, also cause high levels of ANA, so a positive test is not a definite diagnosis for SLE:

Antinuclear antibodies may be strongly present in other autoimmune diseases (such as scleroderma, Sjögren syndrome, or rheumatoid arthritis).

They also may be weakly present in about 20 - 40% of healthy women.

Some drugs can also produce positive antibody tests,

including hydralazine, procainamide, isoniazid, and chlorpromazine.

A negative ANA test makes a diagnosis of SLE unlikely but not impossible. High or low concentrations of ANA also do not necessarily indicate the severity of the disease, since antibodies tend to come and go in patients with SLE.

In general, the ANA test is considered a screening test:

If SLE-like symptoms are present and the ANA test is positive, other tests for SLE will be administered.

If SLE-like symptoms are not present and the test is positive, the doctor will look for other causes, or the results will be ignored if the patient is feeling healthy.

ANA subtypes. Doctors may also test for specific ANA subtypes.

Anti-double stranded DNA (anti-ds DNA) is more likely to be found only in patients with SLE. It may play an important role in injury to blood vessels found in SLE, and high levels often indicate kidney involvement. Anti-ds DNA levels tend to fluctuate over time and may even disappear.

Anti-Sm antibodies are also usually found only with SLE. Levels are more constant and are more likely to be detected in African-American patients. Although many lupus patients may not have this antibody, its presence almost always indicates SLE.

When the ANA is negative but the diagnosis is still strongly suspected, a test for anti-Ro (also called anti-SSA) and anti-La (also called anti-SSB) antibodies may identify patients with a rare condition called ANA negative, Ro lupus. These autoantibodies may be involved in the sun-sensitive rashes experienced by patients with SLE and are also found in association with neonatal lupus syndrome, in which a pregnant mother's antibodies cross the placenta and cause inflammation in the developing child's skin or heart.

Antiphospholipid antibodies. Up to half of patients with SLE have antiphospholipid antibodies, which increase the risk for blood clots, strokes, and pregnancy complications. If a

Doctor suspects SLE blood abnormalities, tests may be able to detect the presence of the two major antiphospholipid antibodies: lupus coagulant antibody and anticardioplin antibody.

As with the ANA, these antibodies have a tendency to appear and disappear. Patients who have these autoantibodies as well as blood clotting problems or frequent miscarriages are diagnosed with antiphospholipid syndrome (APS), which often occurs in SLE but can also develop independently.

Other blood tests complement. Blood tests of patients with SLE often show low levels of serum complement, a group of proteins in the blood that aid the body's infection fighters. Individual proteins are termed by the letter "C" followed by a number. Common complement tests measure C3, C4, C1q, and

CH50. Complement levels are especially low if there is kidney involvement or other disease activity.

Blood count. White and red blood cell and platelet counts are usually lower than normal and, depending on severity, are used to determine complications, such as anemia or infection.

Erythrocyte sedimentation rate (ESR). An erythrocyte sedimentation rate

(ESR or sed rate) measures how fast red blood cells (erythrocytes) fall to the bottom of a fine glass tube that is filled with the patient's blood. A high sed rate indicates inflammation.

C-reactive protein (CRP). High levels of this blood protein indicate inflammation. Like the ESR, the CRP test cannot tell where the inflammation is located or what is causing it.

## Skin tests

If a skin rash is present, the doctor may take a biopsy (a tissue sample) from the margin of a skin lesion. A test known as a lupus band detects immunoglobulin G (IgG) antibodies, which are located just below the outer layer of the tissue sample. They are much more likely to be present with active SLE than with inactive disease.

## Tests for complications of SLE

Kidney damage (lupus nephritis). Kidney damage in patients already diagnosed with SLE may be detected from the following tests:

Blood tests that measure creatinine, a protein metabolized in muscles and excreted in the urine. High levels suggest kidney damage, although kidney problems can also be present with normal creatinine levels.

Urine tests to measure protein levels

Tests for detecting anti-ds DNA antibodies and blood complements.

All patients who show signs of lupus nephritis should have a kidney biopsy to evaluate and classify the extent of kidney damage.

Patients who are diagnosed with lupus nephritis should continue to receive urine and blood tests every 1 - 3 months to monitor their condition. Regular blood pressure measurements are also important to ensure that the patient's blood pressure does not go above 130/80 mm Hg.

Lung and heart involvement. A chest x-ray may be performed to check lung and heart function. An electrocardiogram and an echocardiogram are administered if heart disease is suspected.

## "Treatments: Chapter 4"

No treatment cures systemic lupus erythematosus, but many therapies can suppress symptoms and relieve discomfort. There are also different treatments for the complications associated with lupus. Treatment of SLE varies depending on the extent and severity of the disease.

Four drugs are specifically FDA-

## Approved for the treatment of Lupus:

Prednisone

Aspirin

Hydroxychloroquine (Plaquenil, generic)

Belimumab (Benlysta)

Belimumab (Benlysta) is the newest of these drugs. Approved by the FDA in 2011, it is the first new lupus drug in over 50 years and the first drug developed specifically for treating lupus. Belimumab is a biologic monoclonal antibody drug that inhibits a protein called B lymphocyte stimulator. It is given by infusion in a doctor's office. Most other lupus drug treatments are given as pills taken by mouth.

Other drugs that have not been specifically approved for lupus are also commonly used to treat the condition. Researchers are conducting many investigational drug studies, including trials of new biologic drugs.

Treating Mild Systemic Lupus Erythematosus

Less intensive treatments may be effective for symptoms of mild lupus. They include:

Creams and sunblocks for rashes

Nonsteroidal anti-inflammatory drugs for fever, arthritis, and headache

Hydroxychloroquine or similar antimalarial drugs for pleurisy, mild kidney involvement, and inflammation of the tissue surrounding the heart

Treating severe systemic lupus erythematosus

More aggressive treatment is needed if there is serious disease progression, as evidenced by:

Hemolytic anemia

Low platelet count with an accompanying rash (thrombocytopenia purpura)

- Major involvement in the lungs or heart
- Significant kidney damage
- Acute inflammation of the small blood vessels in the extremities or gastrointestinal tract
- Severe central nervous system symptoms

The primary approach to treating severe SLE is to suppress the inflammation and overactive immune system with corticosteroids or immunosuppressant drugs. Other types of medications, such as drugs to control high blood pressure, may also be prescribed.

## Treating Specific Complications

The major complications of the disease must be treated as separate disorders, keeping in mind the specific aspects of SLE.

## Treatment for Mild SLE

# Creams and Sunblocks

**Creams.** Steroid creams are often used for skin lesions. However, many patients with cutaneous lupus do not respond to steroids, particularly if they have eruptions that are caused by sun sensitivity. A cream derived from vitamin A (Tegison) may help some lesions that do not clear up with steroid creams.

**Sun protection.** Sun protection is

essential. Patients should always use sunblock creams (not just sunscreens) and always wear hats and clothing made of tightly woven fabrics.

## Nonsteroidal Anti-inflammatory Drugs (NSAIDs)

NSAIDs block prostaglandins, the substances that dilate blood vessels and cause inflammation and pain. They can help relieve joint pain and swelling, and muscle pain. There are dozens of NSAIDs.

Over-the-counter NSAIDs include aspirin, ibuprofen (Motrin, Advil, generic), naproxen (Aleve, generic), ketoprofen (Actron, Orudis KT, generic).

Prescription NSAIDs include prescription forms of ibuprofen naproxen and ketoprofen, diclofenac (Voltaren, generic), and tolmetin (Tolectin, generic).

Antimalarial drugs

A doctor may prescribe antimalarial drugs for mild SLE when skin problems and joint pains are the predominant symptoms:

Hydroxychloroquine (Plaquenil, generic) is the most common antimalarial drug used for lupus. This drug is effective as maintenance therapy to reduce flares in patients with mild or inactive disease. Hydroxychloroquine may help protect against blood clots

In people with antiphospholipid syndrome, high cholesterol levels, and bone loss. It is also an important treatment for patients with lupus kidney disease.

Other antimalarial drugs include chloroquine (Aralen, generic) or quinacrine (Atabrine, generic).

Treatment may start initially with high doses in order to accumulate high levels of the drug in the bloodstream. It is not known exactly why antimalarials work. Some researchers believe they inhibit the immune response, and others think they interfere specifically with inflammation.

## Corticosteroids

Severe SLE is treated with corticosteroids, also called steroids, which suppress the inflammatory process. Steroids can help relieve many of the complications and symptoms, including anemia and kidney involvement.

Oral prednisone (Deltasone, Orasone, generic) is usually prescribed. Other drugs include methylprednisolone (Medrol, Solumedrol, generic), hydrocortisone, and dexamethasone (Decadron, generic).

Some people need to take oral prednisone for only a short time; others may require it for a long duration. An intravenous administration of

Methylprednisolone using "pulse" therapy for 3 days can help reduce flare-ups in the joints. Combinations with other drugs, particularly immunosuppressants such as azathioprine, may be beneficial.

Regimens vary widely, depending on the severity and location of the disease. Most patients with SLE can eventually function without prednisone, although some may have to choose between the long-term toxicity of corticosteroids and the complications of active disease. In certain situations (for example, at the start of treatment for lupus nephritis), steroids may be given intravenously for a few days.

## Immunosuppressant Drugs

Drugs known as immunosuppressants are often used, either alone or with corticosteroids, for very active SLE. Immunosuppressants are particularly recommended when kidney or neurologic involvement or acute blood vessel inflammation is present. These drugs suppress the immune system by damaging cells that grow rapidly, including those that produce antibodies.

Specific immunosuppressants. The main immunosuppressants used for treating lupus are:

Cyclophosphamide (Cytoxan, generic)

Mycophenolate mofetil (CellCept, generic) Azathioprine (Imuran, generic) Cyclosporine (Sandimmune, generic), Tacrolimus (Prograf, generic), and Methotrexate (Rheumatrex) are other immunosuppressants that are sometimes used.

For treating patients with lupus nephritis, the choice of immunosuppressant depends on the severity of the condition and the patient's race. The American College of Rheumatology's guidelines recommend:

For patients with moderate-to-severe lupus nephritis (Class III or IV), either cyclophosphamide or mycophenolate mofetil may be used. Cyclophosphamide is given intravenously. Mycophenolate is given in pill form. Intravenous corticosteroids may also be initially given, followed by oral prednisone for a few weeks. Later treatment may include azathioprine.

For patients with more severe (class IV or V) types of lupus nephritis, steroids plus mycophenolate may be considered.

For patients with very severe lupus nephritis (class VI), immunosuppresants are of little help and kidney transplantation is the main option.

Race makes a difference. During the initial (induction) treatment stages, mycophenolate works better for Hispanic or African American patients whereas cyclophosphamide is best for white patients of European ethnicity.

Patients who do not respond to mycophenolate or cyclophosphamide may benefit from the biologic drug rituximab (Rituxan) or possibly caclineurin inhibitors such as tacrolimus or cyclosporine.

Biologic drugs belimumab (Benlysta) is a monoclonal antibody drug that is used along with standard lupus drug treatments such as corticosteroids, antimalarials, immunosuppressants, and NSAIDs. Approved in 2011, belimumab is the first new lupus drug in over 50 years and was the first drug developed specifically for treating lupus. The drug works by targeting and reducing the abnormal B cells that are thought to play a role in lupus.

Belimumab is given directly into a vein by intravenous infusion. The infusion is given in a doctor's office or other clinical setting and takes about an hour. The patient receives an infusion every 2 weeks for the first three treatments.

After that, the patient receives an infusion once every 4 weeks.

Studies suggest that belimumab may reduce the likelihood of severe flares and may possibly help patients reduce their doses of steroid medicine. However, in these studies, African-Americans and other patients of African descent did not seem to respond to belimumab. Additional studies are being conducted to determine if belimumab is safe and effective for these patients.

Belimumab has many side effects. The most common ones are nausea, diarrhea, and fever. Serious side effects may include infections, heart problems, and depression including thoughts of suicide. The drug is very expensive and some insurers may not pay for it.

## Lifestyle Changes

## Staying Active

People with SLE should try to maintain a healthy and active lifestyle. Light-to-moderate exercise, interspersed with rest periods, is good for the heart, helps fight depression and fatigue, and can help keep joints flexible.

## Preventing Infections

Patients should be sure they are fully immunized and should minimize their exposure to crowds or people with contagious illnesses. Careful hygiene, including dental hygiene, is also important.

## Avoiding SLE Triggers

It is very important that patients with SLE avoid excessive exposure to sunlight. Simple preventive measures include avoiding overexposure to ultraviolet rays and wearing protective clothing and sunblocks. There is some concern that

Allergy shots may cause flare ups in certain cases. Patients who may benefit from them should discuss risks and benefits with an SLE specialist. In general, patients with SLE should use only hypoallergenic cosmetics or hair products. Cigarette smoking is a major trigger for SLE flares. It is very important that patients with SLE not smoke and avoid exposure to second-hand cigarette smoke.

# Reducing Stress

Chronic stress has profound physical effects and influences the progression of SLE. Getting adequate rest of at least 8 hours and possibly napping during the day may be helpful. Maintaining social relationships and healthy activities may also help prevent the depression and anxiety associated with the disease.

## "What is Plaquenil- Chapter 5"

## Plaquenil

### Generic Name: Hydroxychloroquine

### Brand Names: Plaquenil, Quineprox

Plaquenil (hydroxychloroquine) belongs to a group of medicines called quinolines.

Plaquenil is used to treat or prevent malaria, a disease caused by parasites that enter the body through the bite of a mosquito. Malaria is common in areas such as Africa, South America, and Southern Asia. This medicine is not effective against all strains of malaria.

Plaquenil is also an antirheumatic medicine and is used to treat symptoms of rheumatoid arthritis and discoid or systemic lupus erythematosus.

Important information

Taking Plaquenil long-term or at high doses may cause irreversible damage to the retina of

YOUR EYE. STOP TAKING PLAQUENIL AND CALL YOUR DOCTOR AT ONCE IF YOU HAVE TROUBLE FOCUSING, IF YOU SEE LIGHT STREAKS OR FLASHES IN YOUR VISION, OR IF YOU NOTICE ANY SWELLING OR COLOR CHANGES IN YOUR EYES.

BEFORE USING PLAQUENIL, TELL YOUR DOCTOR IF YOU ARE ALLERGIC TO ANY DRUGS, OR IF YOU HAVE PSORIASIS, PORPHYRIA, LIVER DISEASE, ALCOHOLISM, OR GLUCOSE-6-PHOSPHATE dehydrogenase (G-6-PD) deficiency.

It is not known whether Plaquenil will harm an unborn baby.

Plaquenil is not approved for use by anyone younger than 18 years old.

# "The Lupus Diet - Chapter 6"

In general, people with lupus should aim for a well-balanced diet that includes plenty of fruits, vegetables, and whole grains. It should also include moderate amounts of meats, poultry, and oily fish. If you have lupus, following a varied, healthy diet may help: reduce inflammation and other symptoms.

Switch from red meat to fatty fish

Red meat is full of saturated fat, which can contribute to heart disease. Fish are high in omega-3s. Try to eat more:

Salmon

Tuna

Mackerel

Sardines

Omega-3s are polyunsaturated fatty acids that help protect against heart disease and stroke. They can also reduce inflammation in the body.

Get more calcium-rich foods

The steroid drugs you may take to control lupus can thin your bones as a side effect. This makes you more vulnerable to fractures. To combat fractures, eat foods that are high in calcium and vitamin D. These nutrients strengthen your bones.

Good foods include: Low-fat milk

Cheese

Yogurt

Tofu

Beans

- Calcium-fortified plant milks
- Dark green leafy vegetables such as spinach and broccoli
- Ask your doctor about taking a supplement if you're not getting enough calcium and vitamin D from food alone.

Limit saturated and trans fats

Everyone's goal should be to eat a diet that's low in saturated and trans fats. This is especially true for people with lupus. Steroids can increase your appetite and cause you to gain weight, so it's important to watch what you eat.

## Avoid Alfalfa and Garlic

Alfalfa and garlic are two foods that probably shouldn't be on your dinner plate if you have lupus. The alfalfa sprouts contain an amino acid called L-canavanine, and garlic contains allicin, ajoene, and thiosulfinates, which can send your immune system into overdrive and flare up your lupus symptoms.

People who've eaten alfalfa have reacted with muscle pain and fatigue, and their doctors have noted changes on their blood test results.

## Skip Nightshade Vegetables

Although there isn't any scientific evidence to prove it, some people with lupus find that they're sensitive to

Nightshade vegetables. These include:

White potatoes

Tomatoes

Sweet and hot peppers

Eggplant

Keep a food diary to record what you eat. Eliminate the vegetables that cause your symptoms to flare up every time you eat them.

Watch your alcohol intake

The occasional glass of red wine or beer isn't restricted.

However, alcohol can interact with some of the medicines you take to control your condition. Drinking while taking NSAID drugs such as ibuprofen (Motrin) or naproxen (Naprosyn), for example, could increase your risk of stomach bleeding or ulcers. Alcohol can also reduce the effectiveness of warfarin (Coumadin) and methotrexate.

## Pass on Salt

Set aside the saltshaker and

Start ordering your restaurant meals with less sodium. Here are some tips:

Order your sauces on the side, which are often high in sodium

Ask for your entrée to be cooked without added salt

Order an extra side of vegetables, which are rich in potassium

Eating too much salt can raise your blood pressure and increase your risk for heart disease, while potassium can help combat high blood pressure. Lupus already puts you at higher risk for developing heart disease.

Substitute other spices to enhance food flavor, such as:

Lemon

Herbs

Pepper

Curry powder

Turmeric

A number of herbs and spices have been sold on the web as lupus symptom relievers. But there is very little evidence that any of them work.

These products can interact with drugs you're taking for lupus and cause side effects. Don't take any herbal remedy or supplement without first talking to your doctor.

## The Takeaway

Lupus affects each person differently. A diet change that works for one person may not work for you. Keeping a food journal and having an open dialogue

WITH YOUR DOCTOR AND DIETITIAN WILL HELP YOU DETERMINE HOW DIFFERENT FOODS HELP OR HURT YOUR SYMPTOMS.

# "Support Groups- Chapter 7"

Being truly "supported" is a powerful feeling that many people with lupus long to have, and that can help enormously in riding out the emotional "rollercoaster" of life with this exhausting and unpredictable chronic illness.

With its ups and downs and flares and remissions, lupus can lead to overwhelming

Feelings of loss and lack of control. Anxiety, anger, loneliness and isolation are common. Many people with lupus say they feel misunderstood by friends, colleagues, and loved ones.

But there is support out there for all with lupus—in the form of "support groups" where people with the disease get together at a regular time every week or month to talk. Support groups happen in homes, clinics, offices, libraries, coffee shops, hospitals, religious institutions and other quiet corners in neighborhoods across New York and the country.

Typically coordinated by professional facilitators, these safe groups can give people—including yourself if you decide to take part—many things.

A sense of connection. Meeting and talking

with others who understand your feelings and concerns will help you fight back loneliness and isolation, and can actually boost emotional and physical well-being.

Coping skills. Get ideas for dealing with lupus, preparing for flares, handling finances, and not just surviving but even thriving with lupus.

Structure. Most support groups meet at regular intervals during the year and can become something you look forward to and rely on.

Motivation and hope. Be inspired to take a meaningful role in your own care and the future you envision for yourself by sharing and listening to others.

Information. Stay on top of the latest in research, trials, and possibilities for new medications as you hear and share news with others.

Friendship. When it happens, it can

provide a potent tonic for helping to normalize feelings and concerns.

1. Lupus Research Alliance formerly S.L.E. Lupus Foundation

275 Madison Avenue, 10th Floor ✤ New York, NY 10016

Phone: 646.884.6000

2. Contact: info@mollysfund.org

## "Best Lupus Doctors- Chapter 8"

Finding the right lupus doctor is very important to caring for you and your illness. Here is a list of doctors, I put together that are well-educated on the illness.

1. Lupus Foundation of America

6700 Troost Ave, Kansas City ❊ (816) 361-7385

2. Brigham and Women's Hospital 75 Francis Street,

BOSTON MA 02115 | 617-732-5500

3. For a current listing of board certified rheumatologists check out these websites: www.ra.org or www.healthgrades.com

For a current listing of board certified dermatologists try www.aad.org

Please contact the office 973.379.3226, or email us at info@lupusnj.org

4. **THE BRIDGE HEALTH RECOVERY CENTER TOLL FREE: (877) 885-9567**

LOCAL NUMBER: (435) 272-3944

5. **JOHNS HOPKINS HOSPITAL**

BALTIMORE, MD 21205-1832

## "What Does Lupus Look Like? Chapter 9"

Lupus doesn't have a particular look. It can cause a rash across your face which has been described as a butterfly rash because it spans your cheeks and nose. This is the only visible physical symptom.

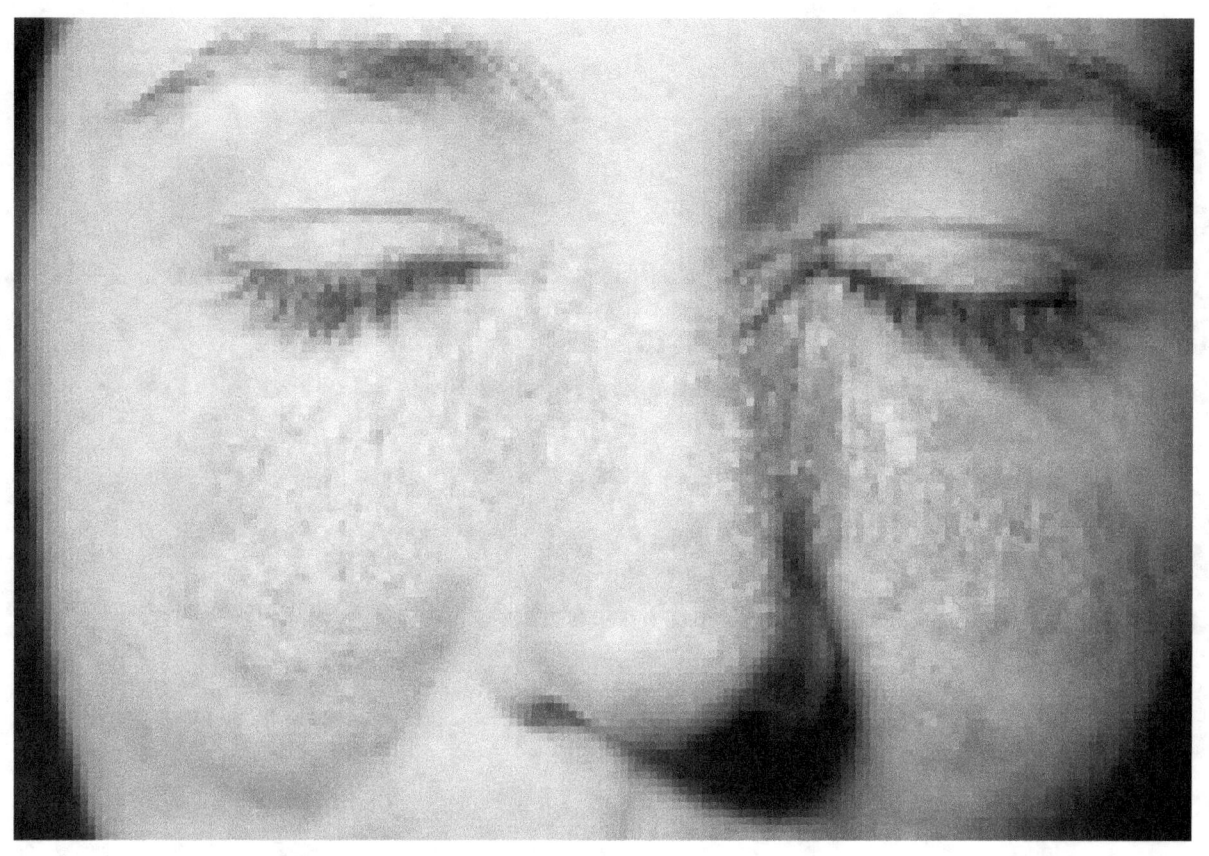

**THIS IS KNOWN AS THE BUTTERFLY RASH.**

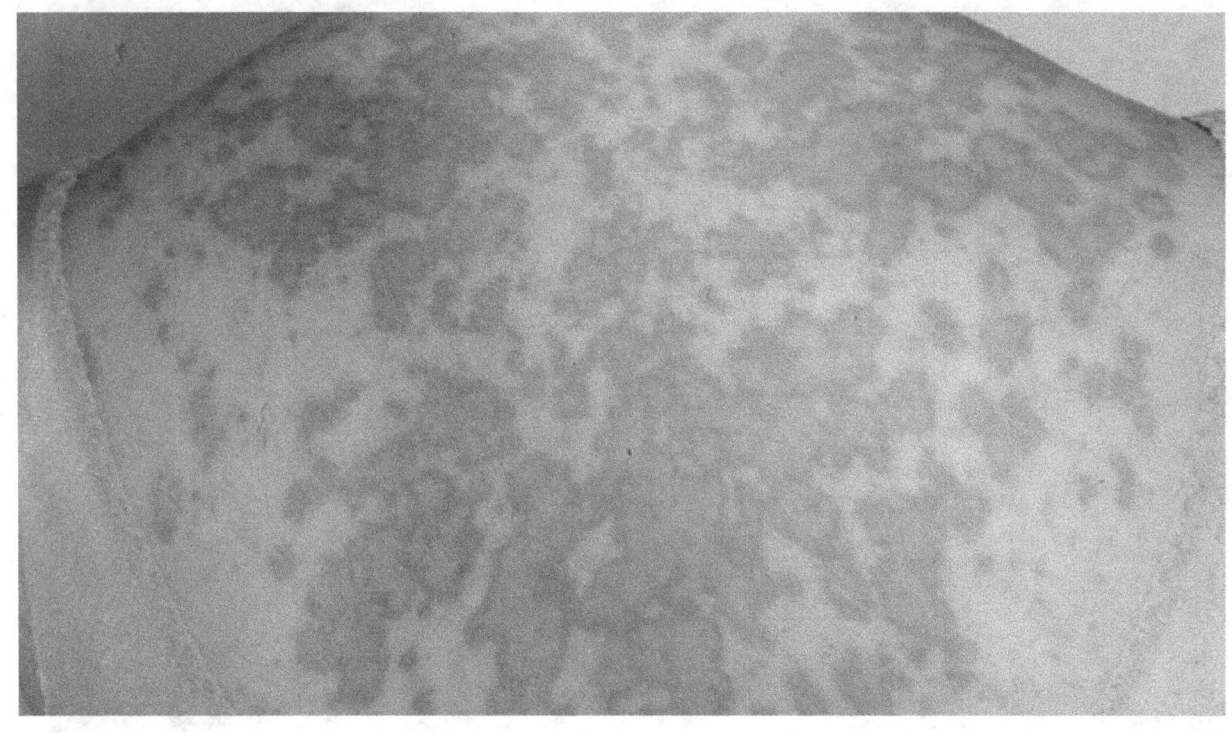

**THIS RASH IS ALSO FROM LUPUS THIS IS WHAT HAPPENS SOMETIMES WHEN YOU GO OUT IN THE SUN.**

www.ingramcontent.com/pod-product-compliance
Lightning Source LLC
Chambersburg PA
CBHW082343220526
45470CB00008B/2619